Fat Bombs

Prep-And-Cook Low-Carb Recipes For Maximum Weight Loss

Nick Rose

TERMS & CONDITIONS

No part of this book should be transmitted or reproduced in any form whatsoever, including electronic, print, scanning, photocopying, recording or mechanical without the prior written permission of the author. All the information, ideas and guidelines are for educational purpose only. The writer has tried to ensure the utmost accuracy of the content provided in the book, all the readers are advised to follow instructions at their own risk. The author of this book cannot be held liable for any incidental damage, personal or even commercial caused by misrepresentation of the information given in the book. Readers are encouraged to seek professional help when needed.

Table Of Contents

Chapter 1 – Fat Bombs Cookbook

Now check these fantastic fat bomb recipes.

Scrumptious Pistachio & Almond Delight

The hit list recipe.

Ingredients:

- 1/2 cup cacao butter
- 1/4 cup raw pistachio (Chopped)
- 1 cup coconut oil
- About 1/2 cup almond extract
- 1 cup creamy coconut butter
- 1/4 cup ghee
- About 1/2 tsp Himalayan salt
- 1/2 cup full fat coconut milk (Chilled)
- 1 tbsp vanilla extract
- 1 cup natural roasted almond butter
- 2 tsp chai spice

Directions:

1. First of all, please make sure you have all the ingredients available. Keep the baking pan ready by lining it with parchment paper.
2. Then melt the cacao butter in the microwave & keep it aside.

3. Keep the chopped pistachio for later use & then mix all the other ingredients in a bowl.
4. It will be best to use a hand blender to make a smooth paste.
5. This step is important. Pour the cacao butter into the almond mixture & start mixing again till all ingredients are properly incorporated.
6. Now spread the mixture into the prepared baking pan & use a spatula to spread it evenly.
7. One thing remains to be done now. Sprinkle the chopped pistachio all over & keep in fridge for at least 4 hours.
8. Finally once ready, cut them into 36 squares and serve.

Some things never fail you.

Total time: 15 to 30 mins

Servings: 32 to 36

Nutrition per Serving:

Protein: 2.2g

Fat: 17.4g

Carbohydrate: 1.6g Net

Funny Scrumptious Fudgy Macadamia Fat Bombs

Mushroom fries bring back a lot of memories.

Ingredients:

- 2-oz cocoa butter
- 4-oz chopped macadamias
- About 2.5 tbsp cocoa powder, unsweetened
- 2 tbsp Swerve
- 1/4 c coconut oil

Directions:

1. First of all, please make sure you have all the ingredients available. Melt the cocoa butter & mix in the cocoa powder.
2. Now this works best over a double boiler.
3. This step is important. Mix in the swerves until well combined.
4. Stir in the nuts & cream.

5. One thing remains to be done now. Then pour the mixture into 6 paper molds.

6. Finally allow to cool & then place in the fridge.

Servings: 4 to 6

My sister makes it every now & then.

Energetic Almond Coconut Fat Bomb

For a eternal experience.

Ingredients:

- 1/2 cup cocoa paste
- 1/2 cup creamy coconut butter
- About 1 tsp. cinnamon
- 3 to 4 drops almond extract
- 1 tsp. vanilla powder
- 3/4 cup coconut oil
- About 1 cup almond butter

Directions:

1. First of all, please make sure you have all the ingredients available. Take a medium sized pan & combine coconut oil, vanilla powder and cocoa paste
2. Now add cinnamon and almond extract to the mixture & blend in a food processor

3.   Now please transfer the mixture from the blender into a medium-sized pot

4.   This step is important. Place the pot on heat over medium heat settings until the mixture is combined nicely

5.   Then place a parchment paper on a small sized pan & pour over the mixture to prepare the first layer

6.   In case you use silicon molds, pour the mixture into them until half filled to prepare the first layer

7.   Now deep freeze the molds by placing them into the refrigerator for about 2.5 hours until solid

8.   Prepare the second layer by pouring over almond butter on top of the first layer, little cinnamon & melted coconut oil

9.   One thing remains to be done now. Place the molds back into

the refrigerator and deep freeze for about 30 to 35 minutes

10.   Finally you could garnish the cup with raw almonds or dry coconut flakes & freeze them

Total cooking & preparation time: about 1 hour

Total servings: 12 to 14

Like never before…

Nutrition Facts (Estimated Amount Per Serving)

14g Total Fat

2.3g Protein

9.1g Saturated Fat

0.6g Sugars

0g Trans Fat

0mg Cholesterol

1.5g Dietary Fiber

26mg Sodium

103mg Potassium

139 Calories

4.1g Carbohydrates

Charming Tasty Cinnamon Blonde Bars

Worth it…

Ingredients:

<u>Second Icing:</u>

- 1/2 tsp cinnamon
- 1 tbsp coconut oil

<u>First Icing:</u>

- About 1.5 tbsp coconut oil
- 1 tbsp almond butter

<u>Bar:</u>

- About 1/4 tsp cinnamon
- 1/2 c coconut cream, cut into squares

Directions:

1. First of all, please make sure you have all the ingredients available. Line small rectangular container with wax paper.

2. Now mix the cinnamon & coconut cream.
3. Pat evenly into bottom of the container.
4. <u>First icing:</u> Whisk together almond butter & coconut oil.
5. This step is important. Spread over the coconut/cinnamon layer.
6. Then put in freezer to set.
7. <u>Second icing:</u> Whisk the cinnamon & coconut oil.
8. One thing remains to be done now. Drizzle over the bars & freeze again until set.
9. Finally cut into bars & serve.

Servings: 2 to 4

Simple recipe for you…

Reliable Delicious Blackberry Nut Squares

Delightful…

Ingredients:

- 2 oz. crushed macadamia nut
- About 1 tsp lemon juice
- 1/2 tsp vanilla extract
- 1 c blackberries
- 1 c coconut butter
- 1 c coconut oil
- 4 oz. Neufchatel cheese
- About 3.5 tbsp mascarpone cheese
- Sweetener of choice

Directions:

1. First of all, please make sure you have all the ingredients available. Press macadamia nuts into bottom of baking dish.
2. Then bake at 310 to 320 degrees until golden.
3. Remove and let cool.

4. This step is important. Spread Neufchatel cheese over the crust.

5. Now in a bowl, mix coconut butter, lemon juice, vanilla, coconut oil, mascarpone cheese, & blackberries until smooth.

6. Taste test and add sweetener if needed.

7. Then pour over cheese. Freeze for about 1 hour.

8. One thing remains to be done now. Take out of freezer & store in the refrigerator.

9. Finally when ready to serve, cut into squares, & enjoy.

Servings: 9 to 12

For those who're ultra fantastic.

Dashing Super Cinnamon Square Fat Bombs

Simple yet tasty recipe.

Ingredients:

- About 1/2 to 3/4 cup creamed coconut, cut into squares
- 1/4 tsp cinnamon

First Icing

- About 1.5 tbsp of extra virgin coconut oil (Please note: Not melted)
- About 1 tbsp almond butter (or you may simply double the coconut oil)

Second Icing

- About 1.5 tbsp extra virgin coconut oil or almond butter
- 1/2 tsp cinnamon

Directions:

1. First of all, please make sure you have all the ingredients available. Begin by lining a container with wax paper or you can use muffin/cupcake tins with liners.
2. Then in a bowl, mix the coconut cream & cinnamon.
3. Pat into the dish or cupcake liners.
4. This step is important. Now please make the First Icing: In a medium bowl, please whisk together the coconut oil & almond butter.
5. Now spread this over the creamed coconut, & place in the freezer for about 5 to 10 minutes.
6. One thing remains to be done now. Now quickly make the second Icing: Now using a whisk, quickly mix the icing ingredients together in a medium bowl.

7. Finally drizzle the icing over the
   bombs & freeze another 5 to 10
   minutes.

Wizard of all recipes.

Perfect Vanilla Coconut Almond Bars

Another fantastic recipe for you guys…

Ingredients:

- 1/4 cup pistachio nuts (Chopped)
- 1/4 teaspoon sea salt
- 1 cup coconut butter
- About 5 teaspoons Chai spice
- 1 cup almond butter
- 1 cup coconut oil, firm
- 1/4 cup ghee
- About 5 teaspoon coconut milk, chilled
- 1 tablespoon vanilla extract
- 1/2 cup cocoa butter (Melted)
- 1/4 teaspoon almond extract

Directions:

1.   First of all, please make sure you have all the ingredients available. Grease a 9-inch baking pan & then line it with parchment paper. Set aside.

2.   Now in a small saucepan over low heat, melt the cocoa butter, stirring often. Set aside.

3.   Except for the pistachios and cocoa butter, put the rest of the ingredients into a large mixing bowl.

4.   This step is important. Now with a hand mixer or something similar on low speed, please mix the ingredients, increasing to high speed, until everything is well-blended, airy & light.

5.   Then quickly pour the melted cocoa butter into the mixture.

6.   On low speed, continue mixing for about 2 minutes.

7.   Next, please transfer the mixture into the prepared baking pan.

8.   Then spread it as evenly as possible.

9.   Sprinkle the chopped pistachios over.

10.   Finally refrigerate for about 3 to 4 hours or until completely set.

11.   One thing remains to be done now. Now freezing it overnight is best.

12.   Finally when frozen, cut into 24 equal-sized pieces.

Prep Time: 15 to 20 Minutes

Cooking Time: 10 to 15 Minutes

4 Hours Freezing

Serves: 22 to 24

Magical taste.

Nutritional Information:

Total Fat: 25 g;

Protein: 6 g;

Carbohydrates: 2 g;

Calories: 227

Pinnacle Cinnamon Bun Fat Bomb Balls

Vintage overload…

Ingredients:

- 1 cup full fat coconut milk (from a can)
- 1 tsp sugar substitute such as Splenda
- 1 cup unsweetened coconut shreds
- About 1.5 tsp vanilla extract
- 1/2 tsp nutmeg
- About 1 tsp cinnamon
- 1 cup coconut butter

Directions:

1. First of all, please make sure you have all the ingredients available. Combine all ingredients except the shredded coconut together in double boiler or a bowl set over a pan of simmering water.

2.	Now stir until everything is melted & combined.

3.	This step is important. Remove bowl from heat & place in the fridge until the mixture has firmed up & can be rolled into balls.

4.	Then form the mixture into 1" balls, a small cookie scoop is helpful for doing this.

5.	One thing remains to be done now. Now please roll each ball in the shredded coconut until properly coated.

6.	Finally serve & enjoy! Store in the fridge.

Servings: 8 to 10

Cooking Time: 15 to 20 minutes

What do you think?

Nutrition Facts (per serving)

Total Carbohydrates: 2g

Dietary Fiber: 1g

Net Carbs: 0,6g

Protein: 0,7g

Crazy The Almond Flour Paleo Bread Recipe

Time for an iconic recipe.

Ingredients:

- 1 1/2 cups of almond flour,
- 1/2 a teaspoon of baking soda.
- About 1/2 of a cup of ground chia seeds or flax seeds,
- 1/4 teaspoon of salt, and
- 4 tablespoons of melted coconut oil,
- About 1 a cup of coconut flour,
- 1 tablespoon of apple cider vinegar,

Directions:

1 First of all, please make sure you have all the ingredients available.

Get a moderate or large bowl & blend all the dry ingredients inside.

2   Now get a separate bowl & blend the wet ingredients separately inside.

3   This step is important. Next, please add the wet to the dry ingredients & then mix very well before you pour them into a greased 7.5 x 3.5" pan.

4   Then smoothen the top, & let it set for about 2 to 5 minutes before you bake at 340 to 350 degrees for about 50 to 55 minutes.

5   One thing remains to be done now. Remove and insert a fork to ensure that it has been completely baked, then cool before setting it on a rack to settle.

6   Finally serve immediately after slicing into 6 or more pieces.

Servings: 6 to 8 slices

Preparation time: 1 to 2 hour

Delicious recipe is ready.

King Sized Mocha Strawberry Fat Bombs

A style statement.

Ingredients:

- 2 tablespoons stevia
- About 2.5 tablespoons cocoa powder
- 2 tablespoons coconut oil
- 1 tablespoon heavy cream
- 1/3 cup of stevia (or per your taste)
- Strawberry Swirl
- About 1.5 tablespoon unsalted butter
- 1/4 cup strawberries
- 1 tablespoon coconut oil
- 4 tablespoons unsalted butter

Directions:

1. First of all, please make sure you have all the ingredients available. Use a microwave-safe bowl to soften the butter.

2. Then allow it to cool slightly before adding cocoa powder, coconut oil, & stevia.

3. Mix it with a hand blender.

4. Use another bowl to mash the strawberries & combine them with heavy cream.

5. This step is important. Warm them up a bit in the microwave (for about 15 to 20 seconds).

6. Now melt the butter for the strawberry swirl & add it to strawberry mixture.

7. Use a blender or whisk the ingredients well.

8. Then transfer the cocoa powder mixture into silicone candy molds or ice cube trays.

9. Add the strawberry mixture to the center & use a toothpick to swirl.

10. One thing remains to be done now. Place the mixture into the freezer for about 20 to 30 minutes.

11.   Finally serve cold & make sure not to keep it out of the freezer for too long.

Serves: 2 to 4

Have you made it yet?

Mighty Blueberry Fat Bombs

Who wants to try this one?

Ingredients:

- 4 oz. butter (1 stick)
- Optional sweetener
- 3/4 cup coconut oil
- About 4.5 oz. softened cream cheese
- 1/4 cup coconut cream
- 1 cup blueberries

Directions:

1. First of all, please make sure you have all the ingredients available. Take out your candy molds & place 3 or 4 blueberries into each of them (depending on the size of the mold you use).
2. Now use the saucepan to melt coconut oil & butter over low heat. Allow it to cool down a bit.
3. This step is important. Add all the other ingredients to the butter

mixture & make sure to combine them well.

4. You can even use a blender to make the process easier.

5. Then if you want, you can add sweetener to your taste.

6. One thing remains to be done now. Pour the mixture over the blueberries in the molds. Make sure not to fill them all the way to the top.

7. Finally place the fat bombs into the fridge for an hour or two before serving.

Alternative Directions for the Pureed Version

1. First of all, please make sure you have all the ingredients available. Put berries, cream cheese & coconut cream into a blender to make the mixture smooth.

2.   Now use a saucepan to melt the coconut oil & butter over low heat.

3.   This step is important. Allow it to cool down a bit.

4.   Put the butter mixture into the blender & puree one more time.

5.   One thing remains to be done now. If you want, add the sweetener & make sure you stir it in well.

6.   Finally transfer the mixture into silicone candy molds & put it in the fridge for about an hour before serving.

Serves: 12 to 24 (depending on the size of the molds you use)

The next big recipe…

Nostalgic Caramel Nut Clusters

Certainly a show stopper.

Ingredients:

<u>For the base of the candy:</u>

- 18 macadamia nuts
- About 1.5 teaspoon coarse sea salt
- 9 pecans
- 9 sugar-free caramel hard candies of your choosing

<u>For the chocolate ganache:</u>

- 2 to 3 tablespoons heavy cream
- 40 grams (about 1 lightly packed cup) 85% dark chocolate
- About 1/2 teaspoon vanilla extract

Directions:

1. First of all, please make sure you have all the ingredients available.

Start by preheating the oven to 310 to 320 degrees.

2. Now place aluminum foil across a baking tray and arrange the nuts on them, with 1 pecan & 2 macadamia nuts in each cluster.

3. You may want to crack the macadamia nuts in half so they lay flat & do not roll around.

4. Then position one caramel candy on each of the nut clusters.

5. This step is important. Once the oven is preheated, carefully place the baking tray inside so that the clusters do not roll around.

6. You will want to watch the candies closely, but they should take about 10 to 15 minutes.

7. Now the caramel should be melted just enough that each nut is secured into the cluster & not so long that they turn into puddles.

8. Remove the candies when this happens & allow them to cool.

9. Then while you are waiting for the caramel to cool down, prepare the ganache to go on top.
10. Use a double boiler to warm the heavy cream until it is almost bubbling.
11. Now stir in the vanilla & then add the dark chocolate and let it melt, stirring frequently.
12. One thing remains to be done now. Once smooth, pour the ganache over the cooled clusters and sprinkle the coarse sea salt on top.
13. Finally refrigerate for an hour before eating these candies.

I use to have it during my exams.

Best Creamy Balls With Jello

You can make this very easily.

Ingredients:

- 1 packet of sugar free jello
- 8 oz cream cheese (solid)

Directions:

1. First of all, please make sure you have all the ingredients available. Now cut the cream cheese into 16 equal squares (2 squares will make one serving).
2. One thing remains to be done now. Then take a square & roll it into a ball & then roll the ball in jello powder, ensuring the ball is completely covered with jello.
3. Finally keep the balls in a plastic wrap & store in fridge overnight.

Total time: 5 to 10 mins

Servings: 6 to 8

Ready, set, go….

Nutrition per Serving:

Protein: 3g

Fat: 9g

Carbohydrate: 1g Net

Vintage Yummy Chocolate Almond Fat Bomb

A little different, a little extra ordinary.

Ingredients:

- Stevia, to taste
- 1 c almond butter
- About 1/2 c coconut flour
- 1 c coconut oil
- 1/2 c cacao powder
- 10 to 15 almonds

Directions:

1. First of all, please make sure you have all the ingredients available. Then melt the coconut oil & almond butter together in a pot.
2. Mix in the cacao powder, stevia, & coconut flour, and combine well.
3. One thing remains to be done now. Now allow it to cool & then roll into 10 to 15 balls.
4. Finally place an almond into each of the balls & stores in the refrigerator.

Servings: 10 to 15

Supremacy defined!!

Lucky Lemon Curd Keto Fat Bomb

Yeah, you can make it in your free time…

Ingredients:

- 1 Tbsp. lemon peel, grated
- About 1.5 tsp. cherry extract
- 2/3 cup Swerve confectioners
- 8 Tbsp. coconut oil
- 1 tsp liquid Stevia
- 1/2 cup lime juice
- About 1/2 tsp sea salt
- 4 eggs, large
- 4 oz cocoa butter

Directions:

1. First of all, please make sure you have all the ingredients available. Place the cocoa butter in a boiler, place it on a stove heat on medium heat settings until fully melted

2. Now you could also microwave cocoa butter in one-minute

intervals to ensure its melted nicely

3.   Add a cup of swerving to cocoa butter

4.   This step is important. Add lemon extract and sea salt to the mixture, stir them well until combined

5.   Then pour the mixture into muffin trays or silicon molds as per individual choice

6.   Deep freeze the molds/tray for about an hour until the mixture has frozen well

7.   Now prepare a mixture of eggs; lime juice & lemon peel in a pan and hand whisk the mixture to blend

8.   Add coconut oil to the above mixture

9.   Then transfer the mixture to a pot & place on low heat settings for about 15 to 20 minutes, stir

frequently (avoid boiling the mixture)

10. Transfer the mixture into a bowl full of ice water and keep whisking the mixture until the curd has cooled down totally (for about 15 to 20 minutes)

11. Now take out the molds/tray from the refrigerator & top them up with curd fillings

12. One thing remains to be done now. Create a third layer of cocoa & butter mixture to ensure the curd filling is in the core surrounded by chocolate

13. Finally refrigerate for 1 hour & serve

Total cooking & preparation time: 1 hour and 45 to 50 minutes

Total servings: 8 to 12

So, what's your opinion?

Nutrition facts (estimated amount per serving)

16.6g Total Fat

60mg Sodium

12g Saturated Fat

0g Trans Fat

148 Calories

1.9g Protein

55mg Cholesterol

23mg Potassium

0.2g Sugars

0.5g Carbohydrates

0g Dietary Fiber

Happy Brilliant Blackberry And Cool Coconut Fat Bombs

I am actually popular among my friends for eating this one a lot.

Ingredients:

- 1 cup coconut oil
- About 1.5 tablespoon lemon juice
- 1/2 cup fresh or frozen blackberries
- 1/4 teaspoon vanilla powder
- About 1 teaspoon stevia drops(add a bit more for sweeter taste)
- 1 cup coconut butter

Directions:

1. First of all, please make sure you have all the ingredients available. Place coconut butter, coconut oil & blackberries in a pot and heat over medium heat until well combined.
2. Now in a food processor or small blender, add berry mix & remaining ingredients.
3. This step is important. Process until smooth.
4. Then spread out into a small pan lined with parchment paper
5. Refrigerate one hour or until mix has hardened.
6. One thing remains to be done now. Remove from container & cut into squares.
7. Finally store covered in the refrigerator.

Grandfather of Recipes!!

Great Mini Strawberry Cheesecake

Different take on this one…

Ingredients:

- About 5 Teaspoon Vanilla Extract
- 3/4 Cup Cream Cheese, Softened
- 10 to 15 Drops Liquid Stevia
- 1/4 Cup Coconut Oil, Softened
- 1/2 Cup Strawberries, Fresh & Mashed

Directions:

1. First of all, please make sure you have all the ingredients available. Quickly start by combining all of the ingredients in a medium bowl & mixing with a hand mixer until completely smooth.
2. Now you can also do this in a high-speed blender.

3. One thing remains to be done now. Then spoon into mini muffin tins, & place in the freezer.

4. Finally it'll take about 5 hours to set, & then you can place them in the fridge.

Prep Time: 5 to 10 Minutes

Total Time: 15 to 20 Minutes

Serves: 8 to 9

I can eat them all day!!

Nutritional Information:

Total Fat: 127 g

Total Carbs: 55 g

Protein: 66 g

Calories: 129

Fantastic Coconut And Matcha Fat Bomb Balls

How is it? Only one way to find out…

Ingredients:

For the truffles:

- 1 cup coconut butter
- About 1.5 tsp pure vanilla extract
- 1/2 cup full fat coconut milk, refrigerated overnight
- 1/4 tsp sea salt
- About 1 tsp matcha green tea powder
- About 1 cup firm coconut oil (refrigerate if necessary)
- 1/2 to 1/4 tsp cinnamon

For the truffle coating:

- About 1.5 Tbs matcha green tea powder

- 1 cup finely shredded, unsweetened coconut

Directions:

1. First of all, please make sure you have all the ingredients available. Combine all of the truffle ingredients in a medium sized mixing bowl.
2. Now note that it's very important for your coconut oil be firm so send it to the fridge for some time if you have to.
3. Same goes for the coconut milk - the thick cream will rise to the top & coconut water will sink to the bottom.
4. This step is important. Now while it's not mandatory that you use only the cream part, please note that your milk should be very firm when you use it so make sure that you cool the can properly or just cool it overnight.

5. Then mix on high speed with a hand mixer, until light & fluffy, then place in the refrigerator to firm it up for about an hour or so.

6. Now while the truffle mixture is firming up, quickly combine the shredded coconut & the matcha powder together in a large, shallow dish. Set aside.

7. With the help of a small cookie quickly scoop form the cold truffle mixture into about 30 to 32 little balls, roughly the size of a ping pong ball or something similar.

8. Then slowly roll the balls quickly between the palms of your hands to shape them into amazing & perfect little spheres, then quickly drop each ball into the coconut/matcha mixture & then roll them until completely coated.

9. One thing remains to be done now. Then please transfer your finished fat bomb balls to an airtight

container & then keep refrigerated for up to 2 weeks or so.

10. Finally these can be eaten straight out of the fridge but taste best when you let them sit & stay at room temperature for about 8 to 15 minutes before to eat them.

Servings: 30 to 32

Whenever you want a great recipe!!

Nutrition Facts (per serving)

Total Carbohydrates: 0,6g

Dietary Fiber: 0,3g

Net Carbs: 0,2g

Protein: 0,2g

Total Fat: 14g

Calories: 123

Delightful The Swedish Keto Buns

Happiness has finally arrived!!

Ingredients:

- 1 tablespoon of whole flax seeds,
- 1/2 cup of sour cream
- About 1.5 tablespoon of shelled sunflower seeds ,
- 2 large eggs, and
- 2 tablespoons of Psyllium husk power,
- About 2.5 tablespoons of extra virgin olive oil,
- 1 tablespoon of baking powder,
- 1/2 a teaspoon of salt,
- 1/2 a cup of almond flour,

Directions:

1 First of all, please make sure you have all the ingredients available. Pre-heat the oven to about 390 to 400 degree F, Mix the almond flour with the Psyllium, seeds salt, and baking powder inside a medium to large bowl.
2 Now add the eggs, olive oil, and sour cream & mix gently for about 2 to 5 minutes.
3 This step is important. Let the mi sit for about 5 to 10 minutes.
4 One thing remains to be done now. Then cut the dough into 4 & then shape them into balls before putting them inside a cake pan & make sure you use parchment papers to prevent sticking.
5 Finally bake the buns for about 25 to 30 minutes until they turn brown & serve when hot.

Servings: 4 to 6

Preparation time: 45 to 50 minutes

Well it is a Grandma's recipe!!

Super Almond Fat Bombs

Iconic recipe of my list!!

Ingredients:

- Stevia to taste
- About 2.5 tablespoons cocoa powder
- 1 tablespoon coconut flour
- 2 tablespoons coconut oil
- 2 tablespoons almond butter

Directions:

1. First of all, please make sure you have all the ingredients available. Next, please melt the coconut oil in a small or medium saucepan over low-medium heat. Set it aside.
2. Then quickly add cocoa powder & almond butter and then mix until you make it smooth.
3. This step is important. Add coconut flour and stevia.

4.   Now quickly place the mixture on wax paper & freeze it for about 10 to 15 minutes.

5.   One thing remains to be done now. If you want an additional sweet taste, you can dip each fat bomb in melted dark chocolate (sugar-free).

6.   Finally in this case, return into the freezer to solidify for another 10 to 15 minutes.

Serves: 4 to 6

Super awesome plus unique!!

Awesome Chocolate Fat Bombs

Stunner!!

Ingredients:

- 1 oz. unsweetened cocoa powder
- 1 oz. walnut halves
- About 1.5 tablespoon tahini paste
- 4 oz. coconut oil
- 1 tablespoon Erythritol or another sweetener of your choice

Directions:

1. First of all, please make sure you have all the ingredients available. Heat the pan over low-medium heat to melt the coconut oil.
2. Then move it into a bowl & add all the remaining ingredients.
3. This step is important. Allow the mixture to cool down slightly.
4. Transfer the mixture into muffin cups or candy molds.

5.   One thing remains to be done now. Now fill about one-half of each mold.

6.   Finally put a half walnut over each fat bomb to decorate.

Serves: 12 to 14

Healthy is a new trend these days!! ? Always I guess...

Iconic Peppermint Fat Bombs

Luxury in its own class!!

Ingredients:

- 4 tablespoons unsweetened cocoa
- 1/2 teaspoon peppermint extract
- About 2.5 tablespoons granulated sugar substitute of your choice (or to taste)
- 1 1/3 cups coconut oil (Melted)

Directions:

1. First of all, please make sure you have all the ingredients available. Put the coconut oil in a bowl & add the peppermint extract and sweetener.
2. Then stir until all the ingredients are thoroughly incorporated.
3. Place half of this mixture into a bowl & set to the side.

4. This step is important. Pour the other half inside of a silicon mold or ice cube tray.
5. Place the try in your fridge while you prepare the second layer so it can start to firm.
6. Now stir the cocoa into the reserved peppermint mixture & mix until well-combined.
7. One thing remains to be done now. You can add more sweetener if needed.
8. Finally if the white layer has started to set, pour this on top of it & return to the fridge at least 1 to 2 hours, until completely firm.

Make me remember the good old days!!

Ultimate Coconut & Matcha Fat Blast

Try this one if you're hungry!!

Ingredients for making the truffles:

- 1 cup coconut oil
- About 1.5 tsp vanilla extract
- 1/2 tsp matcha green tea powder
- 1/4 tsp ground cinnamon
- 1/2 cup full fat coconut milk
- About 1/2 tsp Himalayan salt
- 1 cup creamy coconut butter

Ingredients for making the coating:

- 1 tbsp matcha green tea powder
- 1 cup shredded coconut (Unsweetened)

Directions:

1. First of all, please make sure you have all the ingredients available. Put all the truffle making ingredients in a bowl & use a hand blender to make a smooth paste.

2. Then keep the mixture in fridge so that it becomes hard.
3. In the mean time make the coating by blending the 2 ingredients thoroughly.
4. This step is important. Once the truffle is hard, use an ice cream scoop to make 32 balls & roll them on your palm to make perfect spheres.
5. One thing remains to be done now. Now pot the balls in the coating powder & make sure that they are completely covered.
6. Finally keep in fridge for later use & make sure to bring the fat bombs back to room temperature before serving.

Total time: 15 to 20 mins

Servings: 30 to 32

Relax and enjoy this recipe!!

Nutrition per Serving:

Protein: 0.8g

Fat: 13.9g

Carbohydrate: 1.1g Net

Unique Delicious Vanilla Fat Bombs

Got the idea!!

Ingredients:

- Stevia, to taste
- 1 c coconut butter
- About 1.5 tbsp vanilla extract
- 1 c coconut milk
- 1 c shredded coconut, unsweetened
- 1/4 c 100% dark chocolate

Directions:

1. First of all, please make sure you have all the ingredients available. Place the coconut milk & coconut butter in a pot and melt on low.
2. Now place the rest of the ingredients into the pot, except for the chocolate.
3. Combine & then refrigerate for a couple of hours.
4. One thing remains to be done now. Then roll the mixture into balls &

refrigerate until completely hard, about 2 to 3 hours.

5. Finally melt the dark chocolate & dip the balls in the chocolate. Keep refrigerated.

Servings: 15 to 20

Just got better!!

Yummy Coconut Fudge Keto Fat Bomb

What makes this the best? Check it out for yourself!!

Ingredients:

- 1 cup coconut oil (Melted)
- 1/2 tsp. almond extract
- 1 drops liquid Stevia
- About 1.5 tsp. vanilla extract
- 1/4 cup cocoa powder
- 1/2 tsp. sea salt
- About 1/2 cup coconut milk, full fat

Directions:

1. First of all, please make sure you have all the ingredients available. Take a medium-sized bowl & prepare a mixture of coconut oil and coconut butter
2. Then hand whisk the mixture for about 5 to 10 minutes until

combined well and appears glossy

3. Add salt, cocoa powder, vanilla extract and almond extract to the mixture

4. This step is important. Add Stevia to the mixture & stir slowly until all the ingredients have combined nicely

5. Now place a parchment paper on a small sized pan

6. Spread out the mixture on the pan over the paper

7. Put the pan in deep freeze for about 15 to 20 minutes until the mixture is solid

8. Then take out the hardened mixture from the pan & remove the parchment paper

9. One thing remains to be done now. Cut the fudge with a knife into small, square sized pieces

10. Finally store the pieces in an airtight container for them to last longer & taste better

Total cooking & preparation time: about 45 to 50 minutes

Total servings: 12 to 13

What do you think? ?

Nutrition facts (estimated amount per serving)

15.1g Total Fat

0.2g Sugars

0.4g Protein

13g Saturated Fat

0g Trans Fat

0mg Cholesterol

0.6g Dietary Fiber

79mg Sodium

59mg Potassium

134 Calories

1.3g Carbohydrates

Tasty Pumpkin Power Fat Bombs

Spice up!!

Ingredients:

- 1/2 stick grass-fed butter, softened
- Splenda to taste
- 1/2 cup pumpkin
- Ginger
- Cinnamon
- Nutmeg
- About 2.5 tbsp refined coconut oil
- Clove

Directions:

1. First of all, please make sure you have all the ingredients available. Then please melt coconut oil in the microwave until it is liquid & hot.
2. Then add the butter & whip well with a fork until blended properly.

3. Now keep whipping & then stir in the pumpkin until smooth & creamy.
4. Add Splenda, spices and stir.
5. One thing remains to be done now. Now drop by the spoonful on parchment paper & place in the refrigerator until firm, about 10 to 15 minutes.
6. Finally remove from fridge, roll the fat bomb mixture into 1 inch size balls & place immediately back into the fridge for at least 1 hour.

Leave a mark!!

Titanic Low-Carb Almond Balls

Why not??

Ingredients:

- Splenda, to taste (or equivalent low-carb sweetener)
- About 5 tablespoons coconut oil, melted
- 1 tablespoon coconut flour
- 2 tablespoons cocoa powder
- About 5 tablespoons almond butter

Directions:

1. First of all, please make sure you have all the ingredients available. Mix the coconut oil & the cocoa powder.
2. Then add the almond butter.
3. Mix until smooth.
4. This step is important. Add the coconut flour & the sweetener.
5. Now form into balls.

6.   One thing remains to be done now. Place the mixture on wax paper.
7.   Finally freeze for about 5 to 10 minutes.

Prep Time: 15 to 20 Minutes

Freeze For: 15 to 20 Minutes

Serves: 4 to 6

I repeat… Try it if you want to. No regrets. Right!!

Nutritional Information:

Total Fat: 18 g;

Carbohydrates: 7 g;

Calories: 128

Protein: 3 g;

Rich Coconut Mocha Smoothie

I don't know about you, but I include this one everytime I get a chance.

Ingredients:

- 1/2 tsp vanilla extract
- About 2.5 tsp instant coffee granules
- 1 packet sugar substitute such as Truvia or Splenda
- About 1.5 tsp cocoa powder
- 2 cups unsweetened coconut milk (from a carton)

Directions:

1. First of all, please make sure you have all the ingredients available. In a large cup add all your ingredients together.
2. Then stir well, don't worry if everything doesn't incorporate well.

3.   This step is important. Place in a shallow, freezer safe bowl.
4.   Every hour or so scrape the mixture with a fork.
5.   One thing remains to be done now. Now once frozen, leave on counter until it softens up a just pinch.
6.   Finally pop into your high speed blender & process until smooth and creamy.

Servings: 2 to 4

 Baking does the trick!!

Nutrition Facts (per serving):

Total Carbohydrates: 5g

Dietary Fiber: 1g

Net Carbs: 0,2g

Protein: 3g

Total Fat: 25g

Calories: 234

Elegant The Keto Cinnamon Walnut Power Muffins

Try this my way!!

Ingredients:

- eggs,
- A cup chopped of walnuts
- 2 packets of Splenda (sugar substitute),
- About 2.5 teaspoons of ground Cinnamon, and
- 2 teaspoons of vanilla,
- About 1.5 teaspoon of baking powder,
- 1 cup whole almond meal
- 1 cup of unprocessed wheat bran,
- 12 ounces of soft cream cheese,

Directions:

1 First of all, please make sure you have all the ingredients available. Pre-heat the oven to 310 to 320 degree F & grease 12 muffin pans or cup, or muffin liners.

2 Then mix the cream cheese & the eggs in a bowl in an electric mixer.

3 One thing remains to be done now. Beat the mix until smooth & other eggs, beat one after the other , & then stir in other ingredients except the walnuts and then stir in the walnuts when other mix have been perfectly blended.

4 Finally fill in the muffin pans to the brim, & bake for about 25 to 30 minutes & serve immediately.

Preparation time: 25 to 30 minutes

Servings: 10 to 12

Fresh start with something new!!

Wonderful Coco-Choco Fat Bombs

Wow, that's cute!!

Ingredients:

- 1 cup coconut oil
- Salt to taste
- 4 oz. cream cheese
- About 1/2 teaspoon cinnamon
- 2 tablespoons cocoa powder
- About 4.5 tablespoons stevia
- 2 cups shredded coconut

Directions:

1. First of all, please make sure you have all the ingredients available. Next, please melt the coconut oil in a small saucepan over low or medium heat.

2. Now quickly add shredded coconut, stevia, cinnamon & salt to your taste.

3. Next, use parchment paper to properly line the baking sheet or a shallow pan.

4.   This step is important. Add the mixture to it & press it down to make a solid layer.
5.   Then quickly put it in the freezer for about 18 to 20 minutes to solidify.
6.   Melt the cream cheese & the cocoa powder.
7.   Once melted, take out the coconut mixture from the freezer.
8.   One thing remains to be done now. Now add the cream cheese mixture over it.
9.   Finally return it to the freezer for additional 15 to 20 minutes. Serve cold!

Serves: 10 to 12

Yes, this is famous!!

Quick Butter Pecan Fat Bombs With White Chocolate

Lucky!!

Ingredients:

- 2 tablespoons butter
- A pinch of salt
- About 2.5 tablespoons coconut oil
- 2 tablespoons Erythritol
- 1/2 cup chopped pecans
- 1/4 teaspoon vanilla extract
- 2 oz. cocoa butter

Directions:

1. First of all, please make sure you have all the ingredients available. Use a small pan to melt coconut oil, cocoa butter, & butter over low heat.
2. Now allow it to cool down a bit.
3. Add the Erythritol or sweetener of your choice.

4.	This step is important. Follow it with just a pinch of salt to balance the sweetness.
5.	Then stir in the vanilla extract.
6.	Add a couple of chopped pecans (I suggest no more than 4) into each of the candy molds or ice cube trays you use.
7.	One thing remains to be done now. Pour the butter mixture over the pecans.
8.	Finally place it into the freezer for about 30 to 45 minutes to serve cold.

Serves: 4 to 6

Good recipe!!

Awesome Peanut Butter Buckeyes

Someone is definitely ready for this.

Ingredients:

- 1 cup peanut butter
- About 4.5 tablespoons butter (Melted)
- 6 ounces sugar-free chocolate
- 1 1/2 cups powdered sugar substitute of your choice

Directions:

1. First of all, please make sure you have all the ingredients available. Add the peanut butter, melted butter, and powdered sugar to a bowl and mix together to form a batter.
2. Now if it is too runny & does not seem like it will form, place the mixture in the refrigerator for about 30 to 35 minutes to set before preparing the balls.

3. When you are ready, use your hands or a small cookie scoop to roll your balls.
4. Then each peanut butter ball should be about 2 tablespoons of the mixture.
5. This step is important. Place these on a baking sheet that has been lined with parchment paper.
6. Once you have no batter remaining, chill the balls for at least 30 to 35 minutes before continuing to the next step.
7. Now they will need to be very cold to hold their shape as you coat them with chocolate.
8. Once the batter is chilled enough, add the chocolate to a small, deep bowl & place it in the microwave.
9. Cook properly for about 10 to 20 seconds at a time, stirring around to disperse between intervals.
10. Now it is warmed enough once it will easily roll off the spoon.

11. However, you do not want it so warm that it will not stick to your truffles.

12. Use a spoon to transfer one peanut butter truffle at a time to the bowl.

13. Then roll it around in the chocolate & use a toothpick or fork to lift it out.

14. Next, please hold it over the bowl for a few seconds, allowing the extra chocolate to drip back slowly into the bowl.

15. One thing remains to be done now. Then, place the coated truffle back on the baking sheet & repeat with the remaining Buckeyes.

16. Finally once you are done, let the entire batch cool for at least an hour in the refrigerator before eating.

Best combo ever... Don't you agree?

Legendary Mouth-Watering Jalapeno Popper Eggs

What's so typical or different here?

Ingredients:

- 2-oz cream cheese (Softened)
- 6 eggs
- 4 to 6 tbsp mayonnaise
- 16 pickled jalapeno slices (Divided)
- 6 slices bacon, cooked and crumbled
- About 1/2 tsp smoked paprika

Directions:

1. First of all, please make sure you have all the ingredients available. Hard boil the eggs, cool in and ice bath, and peel.
2. Now chop up four of the jalapeno slices & set to the side.
3. Slice the eggs in half lengthwise.
4. This step is important. Gently remove the yolks & place them in a bowl.

5. Then mash them up and mix in the chopped jalapenos, mayonnaise, cream cheese, and bacon.
6. Make sure everything is well incorporated.
7. Now place this mixture in a Ziploc bag & snip off the corner & pipe the mixture into each of the eggs.
8. One thing remains to be done now. Top each of the eggs with a jalapeno slice.
9. Finally sprinkle the eggs with paprika.

Yields: 12 to 14

Yeah, direct from the heaven; yeah?

Excellent Scrumptious Guacamole Deviled Eggs

Different yet fantastic in many ways.

Ingredients:

- 1/2 tsp garlic salt
- 6 eggs
- About 1.5 tbsp onion flakes
- 4 strips bacon, cooked and crumbled
- 1 tbsp lime juice
- 1 large avocado
- About 1.5 tbsp minced garlic
- 2 tbsp salsa
- Cayenne pepper

Directions:

1. First of all, please make sure you have all the ingredients available. Hard boil all of the eggs.
2. Then mash up the avocado in a large bowl.
3. Peel the eggs once they are cooled & slice them in half lengthwise.

4. This step is important. Carefully remove the yolks & place the bowl with the avocado.
5. Now add the cayenne, garlic salt, garlic, onion, lime juice, salsa, & bacon.
6. Mix until everything is incorporated well.
7. One thing remains to be done now. Place the mixture in plastic & snip off one of the corners.
8. Finally pipe the mixture into the egg halves.

Servings: 10 to 12

Classic, isn't it?

Thanks for reading my book.